Quick & Easy

Stop Smoking

My Experience as a 30 Year Hard Core Smoker

Quick & Easy – Stop Smoking
My Experience as a 30 Year Hard Core Smoker

©2015, John B. Wilson

BullseyeReads@Gmail.com

ISBN 13:   978-0-9854461-2-3
ISBN10:   0985446129

To schedule a speaking event, or group workshop, use the
"Contact Us" page at http://www.BullseyeReads.com, or
contact the author directly at BullseyeReads@gmail.com.

To Mom and Dad
And
To The Millions Who Still
Hold the Future in Their Own Hands

May God bless and protect you all

Table of Contents

Introduction

The Centers for Disease Control and Prevention (CDC)estimates that 432,000 people die annually from smoking; that another 48,000 die from breathing secondhand smoke; and that in all, one of every five deaths in the U.S. is related to cigarette smoking. That's a minimum total of 480,000 deaths annually.[1] These are your family members, friends, neighbors and work mates. This year, if you're a smoker, or are exposed to secondhand smoke, you might join them. If you're a gambler – and you are, if you are a smoker - know that your chances of dying from a smoking related cause are far greater than winning the Lotto.

---

[1] CDC Fact Sheet, *Smoking and Tobacco Use: Tobacco Related Mortality,* updated Feb. 6, 2014, Retrieved January 15, 2015 at http://www.cdc.gov/tobacco/data_statistics/fact_sheets/healt h_effects/tobacco_related_mortality/, content source: Office on Smoking and Health, National Center for Chronic Disease Prevention and Health Promotion

My hope in writing this humble booklet is simply to save and improve the lives of as many current smokers as possible. I'm a past smoker. I quit 16 years ago and I firmly believe that I'm alive today, because I made that decision. What I am not is a medical doctor, or a PhD. Nothing in this book should be construed as medical advice and you should definitely check with your physician before starting this, or any other stop smoking plan. What you will read here is how a hard core smoker – me – quit "Cold Turkey," **without the agony of withdrawal symptoms and without gaining weight.** If you're like me, you've probably used both of those fears – weight gain and withdrawals - as justification for not quitting "just yet." It seems that there's always just one more stressful event on the horizon that keeps us from quitting...just yet. Maybe it's final exams. Maybe there's a problem at work, or you're going through a tough personal situation. Maybe the holidays are approaching and you're afraid to pile on the pounds.

There's a million reasons not to stop smoking...just yet. None of them are good. Be that as it may, you know you've probably used them very effectively on yourself. I did – until I didn't. **Then I quit – no pain,**

no fuss. It was a non-event that might have saved me a lot of problems if I had only done it sooner. But, I prefer to think of it in terms of where I would be now, if I had continued smoking. I believe that location to be the Cemetery. You however, may be in time to avoid both the Cemetery and some, or all of the physical problems I've experienced. That's your decision. Only you can say if you're ready to stop. And you won't be able to stop until you're truly ready.

This will be a short book. I've provided some background that I believe is typical of many smokers my age. It might seem a bit off subject, but hopefully it will serve as a reminder of what our habits may be doing to our own kids and perhaps through them, to our grandkids. When you make the decision to stop smoking, you may be saving not only yourself, but future generations as well. So, bear with me for a very few pages and I will leave you with a method of quitting that worked perfectly for me. It costs nothing, except your time and commitment. It is so easy, that you will feel like laughing or screaming at me. But, if you really think about it, you may realize that the greatest solutions are very often the least complicated.

If anything here resonates with you – if it helps you make the decision to stop - if the plan shown here is the one that works for you, or if something here leads you to design, or adopt any other successful stop smoking plan, I will be very thankful. I mean that, as a fellow human being and as somebody who spent 30 years unconsciously accepting that quitting was impossible.

If you are interested in having the author speak to your group on this subject, in suggesting future subjects, or in authoring a book under the Bullseye Reads banner, please contact us at BullseyeReads@gmail.com.

1

First There was Dad

My mom and dad - God rest their souls - both smoked like chimneys.

Dad was always referred to, by friends, co-workers and employers, as a textile engineer. He was not technically an engineer. In fact, he never graduated from college, or even high school. That seeming handicap aside, there was nobody who knew more about textile looms and he was well known throughout the industry. Dad followed his industry from New Jersey to Rhode Island, to Georgia, back to Rhode Island and finally to South Florida. Wherever he was, he was constantly being approached by other company owners to run their operations. He could effectively troubleshoot, or completely and rapidly dismantle, repair and reassemble the most intricate textile loom. He was even offered a teaching position by a company manufacturing these looms.

When textile began disappearing from Florida, dad was immediately offered new positions, including one in Canada and another in California. He refused both. He had made his last move. Instead, in his mid-forties, he decided to get out of the factories and into the sun. He started his own company, applying exterior roof and wall coatings to residential and commercial buildings. In this new endeavor he was up and down ladders all day, every day. He was a tough WWII veteran with an independent streak, a strong character and a firm belief that he could build a solid, prosperous business through good products and outstanding service.

As he built the coating business, he had his share of setbacks and he had successes. But, it was not sales, hard work, great people skills, or even the economy that made the difference for him. It was smoking. He was literally brought to his knees by cigarettes. He once told me that while in the military, he smoked five packs everyday, of one of the strongest cigarettes on the market. During his middle years, that probably dropped to as low as 2 ½ packs.

At age 55, dad had a major heart attack. That, along with lung problems, left this once robust, self starting, WWII veteran, textile engineer, businessman, dreamer, husband and father with an inability to walk more than the length of two normal house lots (about 150 feet). It was enough to finally make him quit smoking, but in his case, it was already too late.

It would not be long before an oxygen tank was his constant companion. At age 55 he was gone in terms of living the life he designed. At 70, he was dead.

2

Then There was Mom

Mom was a homemaker. No matter how well she cleaned; walls, cabinets, appliances and everything else had that sickly yellowish look that nicotine leaves. She never noticed. None of us did. It had always been that way. The first time I really saw it was when we redecorated her apartment after she died. Even the white refrigerator was cast in a nauseating, thick yellow that was impossible to remove.

Mom lived until age 83, smoking until her final days despite a frequent, hacking cough. She was a tough, stubborn farm girl, and she enjoyed smoking. When she was told to quit, she immediately agreed it was the right thing to do. But, even as she was agreeing, she was already tearing through the remnants of her last pack, foraging for that last, hard to retrieve cigarette stuck in the corner.

When she finally collapsed and went into a coma, we thought it was a stroke. But, it was more. I'll never forget the Doctor, showing us the large mass he found in her lungs. He wasn't sure it was cancer, but it was certainly large enough to obstruct her breathing. The doctor was certain that, given her condition, it could not be removed without killing her and would only add to her discomfort. It was only a matter of hours before she died.

Was her death the result of smoking? I can't prove it. She was 83. She was significantly overweight and she was a chain smoker. My money is on the cigarettes.

She was tough. Whether or not she was tough enough to stop smoking, I'll never know. She never tried. Had she only known how easy it could be, she might have lasted another ten years. At least, that's what I think.

3

"I Can Quit Any Time I want"

As a kid, I had asthma and was in the hospital three times with pneumonia before I started Kindergarten. According to my mom, I missed an entire year of school with asthma, bronchitis and Pneumonia; even spending some time in an oxygen tent. Luckily, according to her version, I also skipped a grade later. What I personally remember from those years, was going through frequent episodes of heavy chest congestion and labored breathing. I remember mom preparing steaming Vicks Vapor Rub in a kitchen pot, placing a towel over my head and coaching me to inhale the steaming mixture as deeply as possible. In part, we had come to Florida because my parents believed that my lung problems were made worse by the cold weather.

We didn't know about secondhand smoke in those days, but I'm guessing that I got a pretty good dose. At the same time though, my mom and dad constantly cautioned me against smoking in the future. Interestingly, it was not because they thought cigarettes were inherently bad, but because of my problems with asthma and what they called my "weak lungs."

In 1965, I joined the Navy. I was 18 and had never smoked a cigarette or a cigar. During the next few years, I seemed to be surrounded by smokers – most of them using the same brand. These were my friends and co-workers. We had great times and I both liked and respected them. Still, I couldn't help myself from laughing loud and often about their smoking habits. I reminded them with all the accrued wisdom of a teenager, that they were nuts to be smoking. They, in turn, probably thought I was nuts. Anyway, they didn't listen. They didn't stop. We still knew nothing about secondhand smoke. My buddies were filling our office and our barracks with smoke 24/7. Given my history at home, I hardly noticed.

Two and a half years later, in February, 1968, I received orders to Vietnam. There were less smokers in my new unit, but still a few. About six months into my tour I tried my first cigarette. I was 21 years old. The rest is history.

After returning to the States, I found more smokers on the job. Incredibly, most of them smoked the same menthol brand as my Navy buddies – the same brand I now smoked. It was easy and very acceptable in those days, to smoke in the office and in the car – just not in sight of our clients.

Smoking at home was also easy. I was smoking more than two packs a day – sometimes three. It was a habit becoming less and less enjoyable as I continued unsuccessfully, to chase the feeling of that first cigarette of the day. I knew it was a habit I could shed at any moment...and since the thought of stopping never crossed my mind, that belief was never tested and never shaken.

For now, smoking was accepted and sometimes even enjoyable. It seemed to have no downside. I jogged regularly and while I got winded, I guessed that everyone who jogged felt the same. I even participated in an 18.6 mile mini-marathon and made it all the way – not last, but in the slower 50%. I couldn't have done that if cigarettes had any effect on me. Right?

I had two boys of my own now and was now giving them the same secondhand smoke I had received as a kid. Like me in my early years, my older son had significant problems with asthma and had more than one emergency room visit as a result. I never imagined any part of that could have a relationship with my smoking. The ER doctors never asked if I was a smoker and never talked about the dangers of secondhand smoke.

4

Living in a Cloud of Smoke

During my 30's, I remember visiting our family doctor for a routine physical. He explained that I had some minor plaque, but it was about the same as anyone my age. I had no idea what he meant by "Plaque," but figured that if it was about the same as others my age, there was probably no reason for concern. I was the poster boy for that commercial that shows everybody questioning everyone about everything, but accepting in silence everything their doctor said. So, I didn't ask and he didn't take it upon himself to explain what was happening.

During the next few years, I continued to exercise moderately, jogging every day. But, although I forced myself, the jogging was painful. I felt like I could never get enough air. Yet, somehow, I managed to compensate by breathing deeper and by running a little slower. I was also losing weight, which seemed to help. I told myself that if I could jog for three to five miles daily, I had to be in great shape.

I devoted a couple of nights each week to teaching an adult education class and it was during one of these sessions, that I first noticed a pounding in my chest – an awareness of my heart that I had never before experienced. I thought about it briefly and then dismissed the event as meaningless. After all, I was in my 30's, running every day and keeping my weight in check. I was good.

At 42, I found my soul mate. Home was a far happier place than ever before. The kids were grown and on their own – both healthy, thank God. I was in the process of writing a college textbook and at work, I had just received one of the most challenging assignments of my career. Things were going well all the way around.

My wife was a smoker, but unlike me, she was content to have two or three cigarettes a day – no more.

We converted one of our bedrooms to an office and I spent hour upon hour there, working on the book. And, I spent hour upon hour there, smoking.

Visiting friends would hesitate out of politeness, but, family members were never too shy to drop a comment about the smell of cigarettes in my home office. I didn't get it. I couldn't smell a thing. Everything was as it had been for my entire life. I had almost completely lost my sense of smell.

But, the smell was not the only clue. A dense grey cloud hung in the air, surrounding and saturating my books, computer and everything else in that room. The health risk of working in that office didn't require testing. One needed only to look through the window to see the difference in air quality from my office to the rest of the house. Spending hours working in that room was tantamount to a suicide attempt.

We had built a very attractive and comfortable front porch and after some discussion, agreed that this should be the only smoking zone in our house. That meant that I would probably be spending more time outside – away from my computer, my book and my wife. For her, it meant that we would have a smoke free home and that she might find herself smoking a bit more, so that we could spend more time together. Even now, cigarettes were somehow dictating our actions and priorities. Actually, they were controlling my life – just as they had been for years.

The front porch became our conversation area and, as predicted, it allowed the interior of our home to take on a never before experienced freshness. We could enjoy both areas. I found myself smoking a little less. My wife was smoking slightly more. At work, smoking was no longer permitted in the building. But, the job called for a great deal of movement and so, there were always opportunities to grab a cigarette. Somehow, the ability to smoke between two and three packs a day remained unaffected. I was still exercising regularly. All was well.

5

Angioplasty – A Wake-up Call

It was a Friday, just after New Years of 1994. I was four months shy of 47 years old, still exercising regularly – still smoking between two and three packs of menthol cigarettes daily. Business as usual.

As I left the house for work that day, I remember experiencing a crushing feeling on my chest and despite it being a pretty cold day(by Florida standards), I was sweating profusely from the forehead. I entered the car, torn in two directions. One part of me said "forget it, it'll pass. Let's just get to work – there's plenty to do." The other side felt a strange sense of dread.

I started the car and pulled out, headed for – I hadn't made up my mind yet. As I reached the first traffic light, I made the decision to opt for my Doctor's office. Ten minutes later, I was there and luckily, so was he and his new partner – a Cardiologist.

After a short conversation, followed by an EKG (Electrocardiogram), my doctor introduced me to his new partner. The two of them seemed very interested in whether or not I had been experiencing any calf pain, chest pain, etc., and if so, under what conditions. When I finished answering their questions, my doctor said that I should go straight to the hospital. I asked what he had found and he replied that the EKG was fine, but that there was a change since the last one. He followed by saying that since I had never before complained about anything, the fact that I thought it serious enough to see him, coupled with the difference in EKGs, demanded a further review. He wanted to do a catheterization to determine the extent of blockage in my arteries (the same "plaque" he had mentioned, but not explained, ten years earlier).

I was adamant in my refusal to enter the hospital at that moment. Our discussion had indicated that the catheterization would not occur until Monday anyway, so why should I go now, alarm my wife for nothing and spend a weekend accruing additional hospital charges for nothing. Further, at the time, we lived less than a block from the hospital. So I refused. They warned me to take it easy over the weekend and to go immediately to the hospital if I felt anything similar to the event that had brought me to their office. While I still believe I made the right decision, I remember that weekend as a very long one, feeling that I was walking on eggs and carefully measuring every minor issue as a possible cataclysmic event.

Fast forward to the following Monday, Dr. Close (not his real name) literally completed the catheterization while I was waiting for him to start. He was one of the calmest, least dramatic and most assuring medical professionals I have ever met.

The Doctor's manner was so completely calm and positive that I was shocked as he delivered the message, telling me I had a 98% blockage in a major artery. Everything that followed that first comment was lost – except, of course, the fact that I would need a balloon angioplasty. This was just before stents became part of the angioplasty protocol.

I knew very little about heart disease, or heart surgery in those days. I remembered when I was just back from Vietnam. I was having lunch with a friend, at a TV station. Suddenly, we heard a man scream with pain. We turned to see him clutch his chest and fall to the floor. He was immediately attended by several people and then transported by ambulance. I remembered a friend of my dad having bypass surgery and I thought about all the talk I had heard growing up about this one or that one who just died from a heart attack. In short, I thought there was a very good chance I was going to die.

When I called my boss to let him know what was going on, his tone of voice seemed to confirm my suspicions. After our phone conversation, I really needed a cigarette.

6

Nothing Works Until You're Ready

A few days later, I sat in a cold, crowded waiting room, completing and signing forms in preparation for my Angioplasty. One by one, I saw patients leaving and walking down a long hallway. As I nervously reviewed the paperwork, I was heartened – but not completely – to see that the medical handicappers (only kidding) called this procedure as having a 3% chance of ending in death. That meant that 97 of the first 100 of us would live to smoke another day!!!

During the Angioplasty, I was in a fog. I was there, but not there – vaguely aware of my surroundings and even able to watch the procedure on a TV screen as it progressed. I felt almost nothing until the Doctor said he was going to show me what it would feel like if I were having a real heart attack. I think he then inflated the balloon a bit more, until I felt a constricting feeling.

Considering the number of people I had seen in the waiting room and now somewhat comfortable that I was among the blessed 97 that would walk out of here, I was suddenly curious. "How many of these procedures do you do in a day?", I asked. The doctor answered "Today, I have six." This seemed like the sudden surge in root canals I had seen years earlier. Judging from his answer and the waiting room I saw that morning, everybody seemed to be getting an Angioplasty.

O.K., that should suffice. I was alive and spent the rest of the day and night in the hospital with a sandbag wedged into my groin to prevent any bleeding from the entry site in my thigh. It was a crappy night, shared with a patient who had just undergone major heart surgery and who screamed with pain throughout the night.

Unsuccessful Strategy #1: The next morning, after the doctor had made his rounds, I was released. My wonderful wife had spent most of the evening with me and was there now, to take me home. After being pushed – inspite of my protests – in a wheel chair to the outside valet area, I got in the car. It was one of the very few times that I was the passenger and not the driver. I'll never forget, as we exited the parking lot, my first action was to look into my wife's purse for a cigarette. I guess I must have looked too weak to argue, because she let me take it...but not before delivering a stern warning that it was time to stop. I promised to cut down.

And over the next several weeks, I did cut down. From 2 ½ packs a day, I probably managed to get myself all the way down to one pack...before I started working my way back up to the original number. Clearly, I needed help.

Unsuccessful Strategy #2: I've always been a believer in "mind over matter," and the placebo effect. Luckily, at that time, there was a great deal of talk about hypnosis. A good friend had just participated in an event that culminated in him walking barefoot, across a bed of hot coals, or some other equally hot and uninviting material. He had sustained only a tiny burn to the big toe on one foot. He had guts and had put his body where his mouth was! I remembered our many conversations and our absolute belief that we could do almost anything if we just believed it enough. We had even discussed the potential to heal ourselves, or grow hair, by having the required level of belief implanted as a post-hypnotic suggestion. If you feel like laughing, check out the back of the Monoxidil or Rogaine and see what it says about the placebo effect during controlled experiments.

So, off to the hypnotist I went.

I vaguely remember the hypnotist's office as pleasant and bland. I remember even less about him. What I do remember is that I was never actually hypnotized (that I can remember). He explained to me that the stop smoking procedure was more conversational and less theatric than we see in the movies.

Bottom line is that I ended up about $100 bucks poorer and smoking my next cigarette before I was less than half way home.

Unsuccessful Strategy #3: Another attempt I vaguely remember was in response to claims that a shot in the nose (saline, I believe) could eliminate the urge to smoke. I remember less about the shot and more about the practitioner's claim that he had approximately a 96% success rate. I was impressed and hopeful. He told me that after receiving the injection, I would no longer feel the need to smoke – not today – not ever!!!

Luckily, I had brought my cigarettes with me, because this time, I didn't make it to my car before lighting up.

Unsuccessful Strategy #4: The strategy to end all strategies was a set of daily skin patches – as I remember, they were contained in small glass jars. The system was quite expensive as I remember – somewhere around $200, with patches containing less and less nicotine as the user reached certain stages of the quitting process. The problem with this approach was with the accidents publicized now and again. Patients would apparently use the skin patches and then cheat by smoking while the patches were active. In some cases, this practice reportedly led to cardiac events. Being conservative and I think logical about such things, it didn't seem very smart to begin using skin patches while there was a significant chance I would end up smoking anyway.

So the patch system remained safely in my bathroom cabinet for approximately two years before I finally dumped them. In other words, I didn't believe I had enough will power to refrain from smoking while I had a potentially dangerous patch on my arm. Wow!!!

7

If I'd Only Known it was so Easy!!!

The different unsuccessful strategies listed in the last section did not necessarily occur in the order presented. It's been a long time. For example, the strategy of "cutting down" actually, occurred many times over many years. My belief, based on my own experiences as well as the experiences of others to whom I have talked, is that "cutting down" is almost always doomed to failure. The other strategies listed may work for some. They certainly didn't work for me. This brings us to the strategy that did work. It started with a decision and with the recruitment of a support system.

While my wife was a smoker, she was only barely a smoker. If I say she averaged five cigarettes per day, that would probably be too high of an estimate. I'll just say it was somewhere between one and five –

normally closer to the lower number. Because she smoked so little, she was less inclined to feel the need to quit. It was still an enjoyable habit for her – one she had proven over time, by the numbers, that she could apparently control. What she did want however, was for me to quit. Luckily, she loves me and she didn't want to lose me to the same fate as my parents.

When I had finally made up my mind to quit, I knew that it would never work if I saw her smoking. I would join her in a New York minute and be back to the races. She knew that it was true. So, while she didn't really feel the need to quit, she agreed for my good.

With my support system well in place, the next step was to establish the start date and to mark it dramatically.

How?

We decided to start on a Monday. On the preceding Friday, I purchased a carton of cigarettes and vowed to smoke every one of them. I wanted to thoroughly hate the taste of them through extreme excess. Whatever was left on Monday would go in the garbage (In the meantime, it gave me another two days of smoking). Through the weekend, my wife continued to smoke as usual. I stepped up my game big time! There were two cigarettes remaining on Monday morning when I left for work. I never saw them again.

About three hours into the work day, I received a call from our Central office, regarding a significant and time sensitive budget issue. While this produced a few tense moments, I found myself thanking God and feeling pretty good that I was able to deal with a stressful situation without running for the cigarettes. I looked at the clock and noted that I had (considering midnight was the actual start of the day) been a nonsmoker for nearly 12 hours.

The next hurtle was lunch. But, this time, instead of running out of the restaurant to grab a cigarette or two after lunch, I decided to take a 15 minute walk. Back at the office, I spent the rest of the day in meetings and found the interactions a good distraction from smoking. After dinner, I walked on our treadmill. We then watched a few TV shows and it was bedtime. To my delight, when I awakened the following morning, I had been a non smoker for close to 30 hours!!! This was really working.

The next day was pretty much the same and I managed to walk around the block three or four times and keep distracted with other issues in between. Yes!!! When I awakened the next morning, I already had 54 hours under my belt.

Then came a travel day – a new challenge. After running to the airport, sitting on a plane for almost three hours and then getting to my hotel, a big part of the day was gone. At the hotel, I ran into one of our crew and took the opportunity to go over some work items with him. But, instead of doing that in the hotel, I asked him to join me for a walk, so we could have time to discuss the necessary issues and get some exercise at the same time. He was a bit of a fitness enthusiast and readily agreed. We walked for nearly an hour.

The following day, after attending a required meeting, I walked another nine miles. This was really getting serious now. I had actually been a nonsmoker for more than 100 hours!

That was a real investment and I felt like the guy who has scraped and struggled to save his first hundred dollars and is not about to squander his money on anything frivolous. I looked at the clock, counted the hours and remembered hearing that if a smoker could go a week without a cigarette, he/she had it beat. Well, wasn't 40 hours a work week? I decided it would be for me in this all or nothing battle with myself. Yes, I had now been a nonsmoker for the equivalent of more than 2 ½ work weeks!

After dinner, I was asked by another member of our crew, to have a drink. While he was a nonsmoker, most of the people sitting at that bar were not. This was another test, but I already had the answer key. After a couple of drinks and conversation, I excused myself and headed for the front door of the hotel. A short walk later, a phone call home, a good night's sleep, an early morning walk on the treadmill – all helped to put more points on the scoreboard. I had now been a nonsmoker for nearly – well, you have the point! By the time I returned home, I was feeling pretty sure that smoking was a thing of the past.

I'll never forget hearing one of my coworkers tell another, "Man, that guy (me) has some will power."

On that day, I knew she was right. I did. The funny thing though, is that it didn't seem like it. At some point in the exercise, it had stopped being an exercise and I had become for real – a nonsmoker.

Was it easy to quit?

In retrospect, quitting cigarettes was easier than I had ever imagined. But, then, I had always imagined it to be an insurmountable challenge. It was not. I could have done it years earlier and saved myself a lot of problems. Better late than never, but best done earlier.

Several years after quitting, I learned that I had an uncalcified nodule in my lungs. After a few years of little or no growth, it suddenly began to increase in size and had to be removed. It was cancer – a fact I had long resisted. I lost part of my right lung, but, thanks to God and a wonderful surgeon, I have been able to continue living a normal life, exercising and remaining cancer free. The early detection of this cancer (first found accidentally through a CT Scan for another purpose) helped to make complete surgical removal successful and to avoid the need for Chemo and radiation.

So, here's a reminder that the danger doesn't stop on the day you quit and that until that day, you are continuing to damage yourself and to produce the conditions in which diseases like cancer can take hold. Again, I'm no Doctor, but it seems reasonable that the sooner you quit smoking, the better.

I also learned - long after I quit – that I have moderate emphysema. But, I've been told that since I stopped smoking, it does not get worse. For me, that means I can still handle the treadmill, run when I want to and participate in other exercises and sports. What a blessing! What a reminder that the best time to quit smoking is yesterday!!! I am also thankful that I exercised regularly as a smoker. I credit that, in part, for minimizing the effects of emphysema. Still, inspite of all this good news, I wonder about the future – especially after hearing of the recent death of actor Leonard Nimoy.

<u>Was it simple to quit?</u>

You bet! It was so simple, that you may find yourself asking why you bought this book. But, remember that the simple plans are often the best. I tried complicated – shots, hypnosis, patches (almost), etc.

and got nowhere. Simple worked. So, here it is. The envelope please. And the winner is: Simple!!!

1. Make up your mind that you no longer wish to smoke – not a pack – not a single cigarette
2. Start thinking of yourself as a nonsmoker. Consider how nice it would be not to be a slave to cigarettes – How it would be to enjoy a leisurely meal at a nice restaurant without running to the door to have a cigarette. Think about all the health problems you are inviting by smoking and how easily your action now might prevent them. Try to reflect on these things throughout the day – maybe for several days. Think about these things each time you start to light a cigarette.
3. Talk to any other smokers in the house and ask them to stop with you. If they refuse, ask them to refrain from smoking in the house, or in your presence. If they refuse, soldier on. Remember my mention of having a few drinks and watching other patrons smoke. When they light up, you light out – have a walk!
4. Open the windows for a few days and let the fresh air reduce or eliminate the odor of

cigarettes in the house. Clean the house thoroughly.

5. Get rid of all smoking reminders: lighters, matches, lighter fluid, coupons, used packages, etc.

6. Pick a drop dead (no pun intended) starting date.

7. Pick the dramatic lead up to that date – mine was smoking an entire carton of cigarettes, but I certainly can't recommend that to anyone else, The purpose for me, was to smoke to excess and develop an intense dislike for the taste of cigarettes.

8. Every time you feel like smoking, go for a long walk. If you have to walk ten miles, so be it. If you have only the time to walk around the block, that will have to do.

9. If you're in a situation where walking is not possible, engage a coworker in conversation. Drink water. Do whatever it takes until the urge passes. As soon as the opportunity presents itself, walk. You are breaking one habit (smoking) as you create a second (walking and health consciousness). That shift in focus is a game changer. Each time

you opt for that long walk, you're becoming less of a smoker and more of a fitness thinker. It feels like magic!!!

10. Add other exercises, if you can. This can add to the distraction you created by walking; helping you to shift focus from smoking to conditioning.

11. **<u>DO NOT</u>** count the days since you quit. Count the hours. The numbers will run up quickly, increasing your sense of accomplishment and making you more and more protective of your gains.

Congratulate yourself
You did it!!!